Syphilis and its nutritional guide

Navigating Dietary Choices to Enhance Recovery and Well-being

Javier F. Williams

Table of contents

Chapter 1: Introduction

Syphilis, a sexually transmitted infection caused by the bacterium Tcomplicationsreponema pallidum, poses significant health challenges, with potential if left untreated. While medical interventions remain crucial, there's a growing recognition of the role nutrition can play in supporting the body's healing processes.

Understanding the complexities of syphilis and its impact on health is the foundation of this guide. As we explore the interplay between syphilis and nutrition, it's essential to approach the subject with sensitivity and a deep understanding of the dynamic relationship between medical treatment and lifestyle choices.

Nutrition, with its influence on immune function and overall well-being, is increasingly seen as a complementary aspect in syphilis management. This guide does not replace professional medical advice but aims to empower individuals with knowledge to make informed decisions about their health. By integrating nutrition into the overall care plan, readers can actively participate in supporting their well-being and fostering a holistic approach to syphilis management.

Throughout the subsequent sections, we will delve deeper into specific dietary recommendations, meal planning strategies, and lifestyle considerations. Our goal is to provide a valuable resource, offering practical insights to empower individuals in making choices that positively contribute to their health and recovery.

Chapter 2:Nutritional Foundations

A sound nutritional foundation is crucial for maintaining overall health and plays a significant role in supporting the body's immune system. In the context of syphilis, a balanced and nutritious diet becomes even more essential. Proper nutrition can contribute to the body's resilience and aid in coping with the challenges posed by this sexually transmitted infection.

1. **Macronutrients:**

Adequate intake of macronutrients, including carbohydrates, proteins, and fats, provides the energy needed for bodily functions. During syphilis infection, the body may experience increased energy demands, making it vital to ensure a well-balanced diet.

2. **Micronutrients:**

Crucial vitamins and minerals play a vital role in immune function. Nutrients such as vitamin C, vitamin D, zinc, and selenium are particularly important for supporting the immune system's response to infections, including syphilis.

3. Hydration:

Maintaining proper hydration is fundamental for overall health. Hydration supports the body's ability to flush out toxins and aids in various physiological processes. Individuals with syphilis should prioritize staying well-hydrated to assist in the body's recovery.

4. Protein Intake:

Protein is necessary for the immune system and tissue repair.. Including adequate protein sources in the diet, such as lean meats, legumes, and dairy, can support the body's healing processes during and after syphilis infection.

5. Fiber-Rich Foods:

Fiber is beneficial for gut health and can contribute to a balanced microbiome. An improved immune system is linked to a healthy gut microbiota Including whole grains, fruits, and vegetables in the diet can enhance gut health.

In summary, establishing a strong nutritional foundation through a well-balanced diet is pivotal in supporting the body's resilience during syphilis infection. Adequate intake of macronutrients, micronutrients, hydration, protein, and fiber can collectively contribute to overall well-being and aid in managing the impact of syphilis on the body.

Key Nutrients for Immune Support:

The immune system plays a critical role in defending the body against infections, including syphilis. Certain key nutrients are particularly important for supporting immune function and can be beneficial in the context of syphilis management.

1. Vitamin C:

Vitamin C is known for its immune-boosting properties. It promotes the production of white blood cells and helps the body fight infections.

Including citrus fruits, berries, and leafy greens in the diet can provide a good source of vitamin C.

2. **Vitamin D:**

Vitamin D is crucial for immune regulation. A decreased risk of infection has been linked to adequate vitamin D levels.l Sunlight exposure and dietary sources like fatty fish and fortified foods contribute to maintaining optimal vitamin D levels.

3. **Zinc:**

Zinc is an essential mineral that helps the immune system do a variety of things. Immune cells' growth and function are influenced by it. Foods rich in zinc include nuts, seeds, legumes, and lean meats.

4. **Selenium**:

Selenium is an antioxidant that helps protect cells from damage and supports the immune system. Including selenium-rich foods like Brazil nuts, fish, and whole grains can be beneficial.

5. **Omega-3 Fatty Acids**:

Omega-3 fatty acids, found in fatty fish, flaxseeds, and walnuts, have anti-inflammatory properties. Supporting a balanced inflammatory response is crucial for overall immune function.

Incorporating these key nutrients into the diet can contribute to a strengthened immune response, potentially aiding the body in managing the impact of syphilis. However, it's important to note that nutrition should complement, not replace, medical treatments prescribed by healthcare professionals.

The Role of Diet in Syphilis Management:

While nutrition alone cannot cure syphilis, a well-thought-out diet can play a supportive role in managing the impact of the infection on the body. Here's how dietary choices can contribute to overall syphilis management:

1. **Supporting Immune Function**:

A diet rich in immune-supportive nutrients, as discussed earlier, can help the body respond more effectively to the infection. Strengthening the immune system is crucial in managing the progression of syphilis.

2. Anti-Inflammatory Foods:

Including anti-inflammatory foods in the diet, such as fruits, vegetables, and omega-3 fatty acids, can help mitigate inflammation associated with syphilis. This may contribute to alleviating symptoms and promoting overall well-being.

3. Hydration for Recovery:

Adequate hydration is essential during illness. It helps the body flush out toxins and supports various physiological processes. Individuals with syphilis should prioritize staying well-hydrated to aid in the recovery process.

4. Nutrient-Dense Foods:

Choosing nutrient-dense foods ensures that the body receives essential vitamins and minerals for optimal function. Whole grains, lean proteins, fruits, and vegetables contribute to overall health and resilience during and after syphilis infection.

5. **Collaboration with Medical Treatment**:

It's crucial to emphasize that dietary strategies should complement medical treatments prescribed by healthcare professionals. Nutrition can enhance the body's ability to cope with syphilis, but medical interventions remain the primary approach to managing the infection.

A thoughtful approach to diet can be a valuable component in the comprehensive management of syphilis. By focusing on immune support, anti-inflammatory choices, hydration, and nutrient-dense foods, individuals can optimize their overall health and assist in the body's response to syphilis. Always consult with healthcare professionals for personalized guidance on syphilis management.

Chapter 3: Foods to Include

Foods to Include in Syphilis Nutritional Guide

In the journey to manage syphilis effectively, the importance of a well-balanced and nutrient-rich diet cannot be overstated. The right foods can play a crucial role in supporting the body's immune response and overall healing process. Here, we explore specific categories of foods that are beneficial for individuals dealing with syphilis.

Antioxidant-Rich Choices

Antioxidants are formidable allies in the battle against syphilis. Free radicals are unstable molecules that can damage cells and are neutralized by these compounds. Including a variety of antioxidant-rich foods in your diet can contribute significantly to the overall health and recovery process.

Vitamin C, a potent antioxidant, is known for its immune-boosting properties. Vitamin C can be found in abundance in citrus fruits, strawberries, bell peppers, and leafy greens.. Additionally, incorporating foods rich in beta-carotene, such as carrots, sweet potatoes, and spinach, provides the body with essential antioxidants.

Berries, including blueberries, raspberries, and blackberries, are not only delicious but also packed with antioxidants. These tiny powerhouses can help combat inflammation and support the body's natural defenses.

Nutrient-Dense Options for Healing

In the context of syphilis, choosing nutrient-dense foods is paramount for supporting the body's healing mechanisms. Nutrient-dense options are those that provide a high concentration of vitamins, minerals, and other essential nutrients relative to their calorie content.

Leafy green vegetables, such as kale, spinach, and Swiss chard, are rich in vitamins A, C, and K, as well as minerals like iron and calcium. These vegetables contribute not only to immune function but also to overall health and vitality.

Lean proteins, such as poultry, fish, and legumes, offer essential amino acids necessary for tissue repair and immune system support. Omega-3 fatty acids found in fatty fish like salmon and trout have anti-inflammatory properties, making them beneficial for individuals managing syphilis.

Whole grains, such as quinoa, brown rice, and oats, are excellent sources of fiber, vitamins, and minerals. Fiber aids in digestion and helps maintain stable blood sugar levels, contributing to overall well-being.

Including a variety of colorful vegetables and fruits ensures a broad spectrum of nutrients. Red and orange vegetables, like tomatoes and bell peppers, provide vitamins A and C, while dark-colored fruits, such as grapes and cherries, offer antioxidants like resveratrol.

In summary, a diet rich in antioxidants and nutrient-dense foods is fundamental for individuals navigating the complexities of syphilis. By incorporating a diverse range of these foods, individuals can actively contribute to their overall well-being and support the body's healing processes. As always, it is essential to consult with healthcare professionals to tailor dietary choices to individual needs and circumstances.

Chapter 4: Foods to Avoid

1. **Excessive Alcohol**:
   - Alcohol can weaken the immune system, making it harder for the body to combat infections. Individuals with syphilis should limit alcohol intake to support their overall health and immune function.
2. **Processed Foods**:
   - High consumption of processed foods, laden with sugars and unhealthy fats, may compromise the immune system. Opt for whole, nutrient-dense foods to provide essential vitamins and minerals.

Potential Triggers and Aggravators:

1. **Stress Management**:
   - Chronic stress can negatively impact the immune system. Support your overall well-being by participating in

activities that reduce stress, such as meditation, yoga, or deep breathing exercises.

2. **Adequate Sleep**:
    - Lack of sleep can weaken the immune system. Ensure you get sufficient rest to promote healing and recovery during and after syphilis treatment.

3. **Hygiene Practices**:
    - Support your overall well-being by participating in activities that reduce stress, such as meditation, yoga, or deep breathing exercises.Regular handwashing and proper personal care can contribute to overall health.

4. **Quit Smoking**:
    - Smoking can exacerbate the effects of syphilis and hinder the healing process. Quitting smoking is a significant step towards improving overall health.

Making Informed Dietary Decisions:

1. **Balanced Diet**:
   - A diet high in fruits, vegetables, whole grains, lean proteins, and healthy fats should be the primary focus. These provide essential nutrients that support overall health.
2. **Vitamin C-Rich Foods**:
   - Include citrus fruits, berries, and leafy greens, which are high in vitamin C, in your diet. Vitamin C is known for its immune-boosting properties.
3. **Omega-3 Fatty Acids**:
   - Include flaxseeds, walnuts, fatty fish (such as salmon and mackerel), and other sources of omega-3 fatty acids. These can have anti-inflammatory effects.
4. **Hydration:**
   - Staying well-hydrated is essential for overall health. Adequate water intake supports various bodily functions and helps flush out toxins.

5. **Consultation with Healthcare Professionals**:

- Individual dietary needs can vary. Consult with healthcare professionals for personalized advice based on your specific health condition, treatment plan, and dietary preferences.

In conclusion, while diet alone cannot cure syphilis, adopting a healthy lifestyle and making informed dietary decisions can contribute to overall well-being. It's crucial to integrate these choices into a comprehensive healthcare plan under the guidance of qualified medical professionals. Syphilis treatment should always be the primary focus, and any lifestyle changes should complement, not replace, medical care.

Chapter 5: Meal Planning

In the realm of health and well-being, nutrition plays a pivotal role in supporting the body's functions, particularly during times of illness. After receiving a doctor's prescription, incorporating a well-balanced diet into your routine can be an essential part of overall healthcare.

Understanding the Role of Nutrition

Nutrition is not a cure for medical conditions, but it can contribute to the body's resilience and aid in the recovery process. For individuals dealing with health challenges, including those with conditions like syphilis, a well-thought-out diet can be a supportive element.

Importance of Consulting with Healthcare Professionals

Before implementing any dietary changes, it's crucial to consult with healthcare professionals.Based on your particular health condition, medications, and individual requirements, they can offer individualized advice. In the case of syphilis, medical treatment, typically involving antibiotics, is the primary approach. Nutrition complements this by promoting overall health and aiding in the body's natural healing processes.

Crafting Balanced and Syphilis-Friendly Meals

When it comes to meal planning, focus on incorporating a variety of nutrient-dense foods. Essential nutrients, such as vitamins and minerals, can support the immune system and overall well-being. However, specific dietary recommendations should align with your doctor's guidance and any potential restrictions due to medications.

Key Components of a Balanced Diet:

1. **Lean Proteins**: Incorporate sources such as poultry, fish, beans, and tofu to support tissue repair and immune function.

2. **Whole Grains**: Opt for whole grains like brown rice, quinoa, and whole wheat, providing sustained energy and essential nutrients.
3. **Colorful Vegetables**: Include a variety of vegetables to ensure a spectrum of vitamins and minerals.
4. **Healthy Fats**: Include sources like avocados, nuts, and olive oil for heart health and overall well-being.
5. **Hydration**: Drink an adequate amount of water to support bodily functions and aid in recovery.

Sample Meal Plans for Various Stages

Meal planning can be adapted to different stages of recovery or treatment. However, these should be viewed as general suggestions and adjusted based on individual circumstances.

Early Recovery:

- Breakfast: Greek yogurt with berries and a sprinkle of nuts.

- Lunch: Grilled chicken salad with mixed greens and a variety of colorful vegetables.
- Dinner: quinoa-steamed broccoli and baked salmon

Mid-Recovery:

- Breakfast: Oatmeal with sliced banana and almond butter.
- Lunch: Lentil soup with whole-grain bread.
- Dinner: Stir-fried tofu with a variety of vegetables and brown rice.

Post-Treatment:

- Breakfast: Whole-grain toast with avocado and poached eggs.
- Lunch: Quinoa salad with chickpeas, tomatoes, cucumbers, and feta cheese.
- Dinner: Grilled fish tacos with cabbage slaw and a side of sweet potato wedges.

nutrition can be a valuable ally in promoting overall health and well-being. However, it is crucial to remember that dietary choices should be made in consultation with healthcare professionals, particularly when dealing with medical conditions like syphilis. A balanced diet, tailored to individual needs and guided by medical advice, can contribute to a holistic approach to health and recovery.

Chapter 6: Supplements

1. **Vitamin C:**

Vitamin C is known for its immune-boosting properties. Including citrus fruits, strawberries, bell peppers, and broccoli in your diet can help support the body's natural defenses and promote healing.

2. **Vitamin E:**

Vitamin E prevents cell damage by acting as an antioxidant. Nuts, seeds, spinach, and avocado are rich sources of vitamin E, contributing to overall skin health and recovery.

3. **Zinc:**

Immune function and wound healing depend on zinc Foods like lean meats, dairy products, nuts, and whole grains can help ensure an adequate zinc intake during syphilis recovery.

4. **B Vitamins**:

B vitamins, including B6, B12, and folate, are essential for overall health and can support the body in recovering from infections. Incorporate lean meats, leafy greens, beans, and fortified cereals into your diet.

5. **Iron:**

Iron is crucial for maintaining healthy blood and oxygen transport. Include iron-rich foods like lean meats, beans, lentils, and spinach to support the body's recovery process.

6. **Omega-3 Fatty Acids**:

Omega-3 fatty acids, found in fatty fish, flaxseeds, and walnuts, possess anti-inflammatory properties. These can aid in managing inflammation associated with syphilis and promote cardiovascular health.

7. **Hydration:**

Adequate hydration is essential for overall health and can help flush out toxins from the body. Ensure you drink enough water throughout the day to support the healing process.

8. **Probiotics**:

Probiotics, found in yogurt, kefir, and fermented foods, contribute to gut health. Maintaining a healthy gut microbiota is essential for overall well-being and can positively impact the immune system.

It's important to note that nutritional support should complement, not replace, medical treatment for syphilis. Consult with a healthcare professional to tailor dietary recommendations based on individual health needs and the severity of the infection.

In conclusion, a well-balanced diet rich in essential vitamins and minerals can aid in syphilis recovery by supporting the immune system and promoting overall health. However, always prioritize medical advice and treatment in addressing this infection.

Chapter 7: Lifestyle Considerations

The guide recognizes that overall wellness extends beyond mere physical health; it encompasses the entirety of one's lifestyle. Lifestyle considerations become the cornerstone of the narrative, emphasizing the importance of cultivating positive habits and fostering a well-rounded approach to well-being. From mindfulness practices to cultivating meaningful connections, the guide encourages readers to reflect on various aspects of their lives that contribute to a holistic sense of wellness.

Incorporating Healthy Habits

A central theme of the guide is the proactive integration of healthy habits into daily life. Recognizing that lasting wellness is built on consistent positive choices, the guide offers practical insights into adopting a healthier lifestyle. Whether it's incorporating nutrient-rich foods into one's diet, establishing a regular exercise routine, or prioritizing mental well-being through stress management techniques, the guide provides actionable steps to empower individuals on their journey to a healthier life.

Balancing Rest and Physical Activity

The delicate equilibrium between rest and physical activity emerges as a crucial focal point. Emphasizing the symbiotic relationship between quality sleep and regular exercise, the guide advocates for a balanced approach. Understanding that adequate rest is essential for recovery and regeneration, while physical activity contributes to overall vitality, the guide provides guidance on striking the right balance tailored to individual needs and preferences.

Nutritional Guide

In tandem with lifestyle considerations, the guide presents a detailed nutritional guide that goes beyond the basics of sustenance. It explores the intricate relationship between nutrition and health, offering insights into the importance of macronutrients, micronutrients, and hydration. The nutritional guide aims to empower readers with the knowledge to make informed dietary choices that support their immune system and overall well-being, creating a foundation for a resilient and healthy life.

Synergy of Health and Nutrition

The guide underscores the intrinsic connection between health and nutrition, highlighting how a well-nourished body is better equipped to resist infections, including syphilis. By interweaving syphilis awareness with nutritional guidance, the guide takes a unique approach to holistic health. It serves as a roadmap for individuals to understand not only the complexities of syphilis but also how nutritional choices play a pivotal role in fortifying the body against various health challenges.

"Syphilis and Nutrition" emerges as a holistic guide that transcends traditional health literature. It seamlessly weaves together vital components of syphilis awareness, lifestyle considerations, and nutritional guidance. The guide becomes a beacon for those seeking a comprehensive approach to wellness, encouraging individuals to embrace the interconnectedness of their health. By providing knowledge and practical strategies, the guide empowers readers to navigate the intricate tapestry of syphilis and nutrition, leading them towards a path of resilience, vitality, and holistic well-being.

Chapter 8: Consultation with Healthcare Professionals

Understanding Syphilis: A Complex Landscape

Comprehensive insights into syphilis transmission, symptoms, and potential complications form the foundation for informed healthcare decisions. Healthcare professionals play a crucial role in educating individuals about the intricacies of this infection.

Diagnosis and Testing: The Gateway to Informed Care

Healthcare professionals employ various diagnostic tools, including blood tests and physical examinations, to confirm syphilis. Timely and accurate diagnosis is essential for initiating prompt treatment and preventing further complications.

Tailored Treatment Plans: Addressing Individual Needs

Healthcare professionals develop personalized treatment plans based on the stage of syphilis, overall health, and potential coexisting conditions. Collaborative decision-making between the individual and healthcare provider ensures optimal outcomes.

Navigating Psychological Aspects: The Role of Healthcare Professionals

The emotional impact of a syphilis diagnosis should not be underestimated. Healthcare professionals offer invaluable support, addressing concerns, and guiding individuals through the psychological aspects of living with syphilis.

Sexual Health Education and Prevention Strategies

Healthcare consultations provide a platform for educating individuals about safe sexual practices, preventing transmission, and the importance of partner communication. This proactive approach contributes to both individual and public health.

Monitoring and Follow-Up: A Continuous Healthcare Journey

Regular check-ups and follow-up appointments are integral components of syphilis management. Healthcare professionals monitor treatment progress, assess for potential complications, and adapt care plans as needed.

Collaboration with a Multidisciplinary Team

Syphilis management often involves collaboration among various healthcare professionals, including infectious disease specialists, primary care physicians, and mental health professionals. This multidisciplinary approach ensures a comprehensive and holistic care strategy.

Addressing Stigma and Fostering Supportive Healthcare Environments

Healthcare professionals play a pivotal role in combating stigma associated with syphilis. Creating supportive and non-judgmental healthcare environments encourages open communication and fosters trust between patients and providers.

Educating Communities: The Role of Healthcare Advocacy

Beyond individual consultations, healthcare professionals contribute to community education and awareness campaigns. By disseminating accurate information, they empower communities to make informed decisions about sexual health.

Empowering Through Consultation

In conclusion, consultations with healthcare professionals are instrumental in navigating the complexities of syphilis. From diagnosis and treatment to ongoing care and community education, the expertise of healthcare providers forms the cornerstone of effective syphilis management. By fostering open communication and collaboration, individuals can embark on a journey toward better health, supported by a knowledgeable and empathetic healthcare team.

Chapter 9: Addressing Common Queries on Syphilis and Diet

1.Impact of diet on syphilis progression:

A balanced diet rich in vitamins and minerals is essential for supporting the immune system. Adequate nutrition can help the body respond more effectively to infections, potentially influencing the progression of syphilis. However, diet alone cannot replace medical treatment, and consulting with a healthcare professional is crucial.

2: **Foods to include in the diet:**

- **Vitamin C-rich foods**: Citrus fruits, strawberries, and bell peppers contain vitamin C, which is known to support the immune system.

- **Leafy greens and vegetables**: These provide essential nutrients and antioxidants that contribute to overall health.
- **Lean proteins**: Incorporating sources like poultry, fish, and tofu can aid in tissue repair and immune function.

3.Foods to avoid:

While there is no specific list of foods to avoid for syphilis, individuals with syphilis may benefit from avoiding excessive alcohol and tobacco use. These substances can weaken the immune system and hinder the body's ability to fight infections

5. Managing symptoms with diet:

Certain symptoms of syphilis, such as skin rashes and sores, may benefit from a diet rich in foods with anti-inflammatory properties. Including omega-3 fatty acids found in fish, flaxseeds, and walnuts may help alleviate inflammation

6. Hydration and overall health:

Staying hydrated is crucial for general health and can support the body's ability to recover from infections. Drinking an adequate amount of water helps flush out toxins and supports various bodily functions.

7. **Importance of medical treatment**:

It is crucial to emphasize that while a healthy diet can complement overall well-being, medical treatment remains the cornerstone for managing syphilis. Antibiotics prescribed by healthcare professionals are necessary to effectively eliminate the infection and prevent complications.:

In summary, while diet plays a supportive role in overall health, it cannot replace medical treatment for syphilis. A balanced diet, rich in essential nutrients, can contribute to a robust immune system and may aid in the body's ability to combat infections. However, individuals should always consult with healthcare professionals for proper diagnosis, treatment, and guidance on maintaining a healthy lifestyle.

Chapter 10: Conclusion

The conclusion of the discourse on syphilis emphasizes the significance of education and awareness. Informed individuals are better equipped to recognize the symptoms, understand transmission dynamics, and engage in preventive practices. Education becomes a cornerstone in breaking the cycle of transmission and reducing the stigma associated with syphilis.

Preventive measures play a pivotal role in addressing the prevalence of syphilis. Safe sexual practices, including the consistent use of condoms and regular testing, are integral components of preventing the spread of the infection. Public health campaigns and initiatives must focus on promoting these measures to empower individuals and communities in safeguarding their sexual health.

Advancements in medical research and treatment options contribute significantly to the evolving landscape of syphilis management. The conclusion of discussions on syphilis highlights the importance of continued research, vaccine development, and accessible healthcare services. This not only aids in better understanding the infection but also enhances the effectiveness of treatment strategies.

Addressing social and cultural factors is paramount in the conclusion of syphilis discussions. Destigmatizing the infection fosters an environment where individuals are more likely to seek testing and treatment. Moreover, understanding the socio-cultural contexts that contribute to the spread of syphilis allows for tailored interventions that resonate with specific communities.

The role of healthcare infrastructure and accessibility cannot be overstated in the conclusion of syphilis discussions. Access to affordable and comprehensive healthcare services ensures timely diagnosis and treatment, reducing the long-term impact of syphilis on individuals and communities. Efforts should be directed toward improving healthcare systems globally to bridge existing gaps in access.

In conclusion, the discourse on syphilis encompasses a spectrum of considerations, from individual awareness to global healthcare policies. Empowering individuals through education, promoting preventive measures, embracing medical advancements, addressing social factors, and enhancing healthcare accessibility are key components of effectively managing syphilis. The conclusion, therefore, underscores the collective responsibility of individuals, healthcare professionals, and policymakers in fostering a world where syphilis is understood, prevented, and treated with compassion and efficiency.

www.ingramcontent.com/pod-product-compliance
Lightning Source LLC
Chambersburg PA
CBHW070746260726
48660CB00007B/3003